THE BRONX STREET KID

Into Twelve Step Recovery

Richard Kane

authorHOUSE®

AuthorHouse™
1663 Liberty Drive
Bloomington, IN 47403
www.authorhouse.com
Phone: 1-800-839-8640

First published by AuthorHouse 7/23/2009

ISBN: 978-1-4490-0268-8 (sc)
ISBN: 978-1-4490-0269-5 (hc)

Library of Congress Control Number: 2009906635

Printed in the United States of America
Bloomington, Indiana

This book is printed on acid-free paper.

1. Looking Back

March, 11 2001

Around this time of the year, in 1985 I just got out of the Bergen county jail, I've been in for 16 or 17 months for a parole violation.

At that time I was heavy into the Irish politics "up the republic". I strongly supported the IRA and their views. I used to hate Margaret Thatcher, I blamed her for the death of the 10 Hunger Strikers in 1981 Bobby Sands being the first. I also marched for Joe Doherty the IRA man held in the MCC. At that time right after I got out of jail I went on that last big drunk. It seems that I always drank more around that time of the year because of St. Patrick's day. I ended up getting arrested for making threats against the president of the United States who at that time was Ronald Reagan. I hated him back then but then I was a very sick person. Well anyway I had a look a like pistol on the train and a cop over heard me talking about killing the president. I was arrested and the FBI was called and interviewed me I was let go cause the pistol was fake and the big drunk started again. It went till April 25 1985.

I put the plug in the jug in Woonsocket RI My mother had sent me there to live with my younger brother because of the Regan incident. I got sober there I joined my first home group. The Woonsocket Friday night group I made a lot of friends and got active. I stayed there till 1988 until I moved back to Paramus NJ to my mother's house. I stayed there for 2 years I went to lots of meetings I had 3 home groups all in Bergenfield I had the Bergenfield central Sunday, the new bridge Thursday night, and the Bergenfield young at heart group which I helped start. I went with Dot Murphy she had a great saying "Screw guilt" she was great, lots of sobriety. I kept the plug in the jug for 12 years and then I took it out in July of 1997. Tonight I am once again sober and in recovery just under 9 months and I am grateful for the chance to stay sober again.

Today I am going through the worst time of my life, It is also the time in my life I learned the most. I have hepatitis c and I am on interferon its absolute torture. From this I learned about my higher power, which I have gotten much closer to. I go to 3 meetings a day most of the time and I have learned a lot about my self. I make coffee again, have a home group, and also have and use a sponsor. All of this has helped me to clean house right out of the Big Book, Chapter 5 How it Works, I didn't do that when I had 12 years. It has made a big difference in my life I am grateful to God and to 12 step programs for saving my life. I am grateful too for having the hepatitis c virus, I started on the treatment almost the same time I came back into recovery June 20 2001. I started on the interferon in July it appears to be working real well for me I am what they call "in remission" and I only have 2 more months to complete this treatment. I thank God, and all my friends at the Sahara club in Hackensack NJ, as I said I go to 3 meetings a day there, I could have never handled this hep c virus by myself. For me to drink with my liver disease is to die , so once again thanks too all my friends at the sober mass in Closter NJ, for praying for me in my battle with the hep c virus I will never forget your prayers and support.

Rich K.
Home Group Sahara
Club
Hackensack NJ

To God: I thank you for my sobriety. I have been sober since June 2001. I am grateful for all my blessings. I am in remission from hepatitis C for more than five years. I have gotten a lot better with my colitis and my skin condition. The more I learn to trust you and your guidance, the better I get. I am working again. I have no problem paying my bills. I trust the future. I believe in you. Your plan is better than mine. I had no goals for most of my life. I drifted around. I was never really lost because I had nowhere to go. I have spent most of my life afraid of people. I kept people away. I have made progress in this area. God, You know better than I what I went through as a child. The physical beatings, the neglect, the sexual abuse; I got kicked around by life pretty good. I am a survivor. I learned how to hide my feelings. I had no plans for my life. Trouble seemed to follow me wherever I went. Of course it would because . I am the problem; no matter what I tried, I couldn't get away from me. I have prayed to you for years to help me to see the good in myself, to accept that I am worthwhile. I prayed about my sexuality; I prayed for the strength to realize it is a gift. It is good and God-given. I thank you for sticking with me, Rich Kane, the Bronx street kid, the dead-end kid, the jailbird, and the drunk. I am all right. I live in the now. I have learned to forgive all people who did harm to me. I ask Jesus to forgive me. I have forgiven myself. You are the force in the universe. You know me better than I know myself. I turn over whatever I can of my life to you. I do the best I can; when I do it, there is more that has to be done. I would hope one day, if it is your will, that I can have companionship with a woman. I will wait patiently on the Lord. All things are possible through God who strengthens me. You know all I have been doing, group therapy, 12 step Meetings the recovery retreats, and the Friday night meeting for sexual abuse survivors. We do have a plan. I have been sticking to my end. Your will, not mine, be done. I hope the progress I made pleases you. I do need to make more progress on some small habits. Thank you, holy Father. Your son, Richard Kane.

My name is Richard Kane. I was born on June 5, 1957 in New York City. My father's name is Harold Kane. My mother's name is Catherine Gillis. We lived in the Bronx on West 170th Street and Merriam Avenue. They call it the Highbridge section of the Bronx.

I am going over this stuff again to help me in my recovery program. It is my life story. I am telling it the best I can remember it. I grew up in a violent, alcoholic home. My mom worked at night and my father hung out in the bars on Ogden Avenue. My sister took care of us. She was only about a year or two older than me. We had very little supervision. I got many beatings for numerous years from my father. I hung out in the streets. I was always getting hurt. I ended up in the hospital a lot. I had a lot of energy and I was wild. I liked the Bronx. I had a fair amount of friends. We played ball and all that kind of stuff.

I started getting in trouble when I was very young. I was arrested a few times for shoplifting when I was less than ten years old. I was afraid of my father, so I would run away. I rarely hung around our apartment. My friends and I used to go down by the Harlem River. We would play under the bridges and we would swim in the river. One time, I was on my way down to the river when I ran into this man. He was friendly. He gave me some fireworks. I was very young, less than ten years old. He talked me into taking off my pants, and he did something to me. I didn't know what it meant at the time. It did hurt me a little. Somehow I know it was wrong. It only happened once. I never saw this person again, so I never said anything to anyone. I knew if I told my family, my father would blame me, and then beat me. I tried to make believe it never happened. I have recently begun to deal with it. I wrote to a priest about it and he said the man stole my innocence. This thing has haunted me off and on. As I got older, I realized what it meant. I had shame. I blamed myself. I felt guilty about it. How could I let such a thing happen?

We moved out of the Bronx in 1967 and went to Bergenfield. There were a lot of problems there. My home life wasn't good. My father still hung out in the bars. He was never around. When he was, I wished he wasn't. He was crazy. He was a marine and he fought in World War II. He worked in the post office.Mostly I remember he was a violent man. I feared him so I hardly ever talked to him. Bergenfield was no different than the Bronx. As far as my family life was concerned, the beatings continued to happen. Some were worse than others. The beds had to be made in perfect Marine Corps style so my father could bounce a quarter off them. If it didn't bounce high enough, I got a beating. The same thing applied to the clothes in the drawers. If they weren't folded the right way, I got a beating. I do remember getting a drawer smashed over my head. I also remember a beating with hedge clippers like it was yesterday. I was maybe ten or eleven when it happened, in Bergenfield, in the living room. I was suppose to be trimming the bushes but I went to play baseball with my friends instead. It began to rain, so I went home. When I got there, the old man was waiting. He went crazy. He had the hedge clippers in his hand; I had left them outside. He beat me on the head with them. I wasn't allowed to cry, so I didn't. Maybe he would have killed me that day. My sister was there, and she started to cry and begged him to stop, and he did. He always liked my sister. I got sent to bed with no supper. When I went to get up later, the pillowcase was stuck to my head from the dried blood. Nothing was ever said about the incident. That's the way it was in my home. The family business stayed in the home. It seemed like a normal family to me. You learn to live with it.

As I said, I'm not placing blame. This is to give me a better understanding.

My 12 step program tells me I am responsible for my recovery, and this is part of it. I was always a nervous, uptight person; as far back as I can remember. I have been in trouble my whole life. I acted out, as it's called today. I was very angry as a teenager. I also began my drinking when I was ten or eleven. I started to drink in Bergenfield. I hung out in Foster Village at the bowling alley. Mostly I would get drunk on the weekends. We used to go to the dances. I was always drunk and looking for trouble. I was in a lot of fights. Sometimes I would beat people up and sometimes I would get beaten up. I hung out with a crew of guys. We stole cars. We committed burglaries. We got into fights. All the cops knew us. I started getting arrested a lot for burglaries. I went to Juvenile Hall; I was a regular there. I got sent away for the first time at fifteen. I did eighteen months at this place in Pennsylvania. It did bother me at first, but I got used to it. When I got out, I went back to drinking and hanging out. I loved drinking and I drank almost every day. I was on probation but I didn't give a damn. I did whatever I wanted. I thought life was a joke. I hated myself and I hated life. I just wanted to stay drunk all the time. I had a lot of run-ins with the police and some fights with them. Jack Moore and I used to fight all the time; he was a Bergenfield cop. Most of my drinking happened in the '70s and '80s. Looking back, I was full of fear, self-pity, and self-hatred, and I had a ton of resentment. I didn't know any of this back then. I do now, thanks to recovery. I have been in 12 step programs since I was eighteen, not by choice. The courts sent me to A.R.P in Hackensack, and I had to go to meetings. I always went drunk; I had a bad attitude and I didn't give a damn. I was in jail all the time. I have been in the Bergen County Jail a lot; I would say between thirty and fifty times. I am not really sure. I have also been at the Bergen Pines Hospital nut ward on the ninth floor because of my drinking my violence and all of my crimes. I got two five-year sentences for burglaries. I was drunk when I did them. I did my state time in Jersey. Being a drunk and a loser and a troublemaker was all I knew. My mom divorced my father, sold the house, got remarried, and moved. I ended up sleeping in the parks in Bergen Field. I was a drunk and I had no self-esteem. I lived in the streets because of the way I acted. People didn't want me around. I drank all the time. I got sicker and sicker. I got the shakes; sometimes I had the DTs. I was sad and lonely; I felt unloved and unwanted. I knew I hated myself. I had my chance to do something about my problems. I have been to rehab. I went to Turning Point, Straight and Narrow, and building 4 at Bergen Pines. As the years went by, my drinking got worse. I could drink over half a gallon of vodka daily; I was proud of that. I did crazy things when I was drunk. I wanted to be a tough guy. I got sentenced to ten months on Riker's Island;. I got into a fight with a cop in NYC. I was in a blackout. I got arrested for assault and being drunk. Rikers Island wasn't that bad. I even got drunk while I was there. I looked up to men of violence. I looked up to the Irish Republican Army. I really respected them. I looked up to Bobby Sands and the ten hunger strikers.. Sands was the first to die. I also looked up to other Irish gangsters, such as Mickey Featherstone and Jimmy Coonan; they were called the Westies. I also looked up to Mad Dog Sullivan and Trigger Burke. I read about these people and I wanted to be like them. I also looked up to the Hell's Angels motorcycle club. I thought it was cool to be violent. In 1985, I pulled one of my crazy, stupid stunts. I was arrested in NYC for threatening the president of the United States. I was drunk and in a blackout. I thought it was funny, but no one else did. I ended up in Rhode Island with my brother. I got drunk a few times up there. Who knew this was about to change?

I stopped drinking in Woonsocket, Rhode Island on April 25, 1985 and began to go to meetings. I joined a home group. I went out speaking. I made a start on recovery. I got a job. I got my own place and I went to a lot of meetings. I began to get better. I never had a sponsor and I never read *The Big Book*. I stayed up there two and a half years before I moved back to New Jersey. I stayed with my mom for almost three years. I still wasn't drinking. I was going to a lot of meetings. I still didn't have a sponsor. I was still very angry. I got into fights. I joined a motorcycle club. I was a Desperado—that was the name of the gang I rode with. As I said, I never had a- sponsor and I never worked the steps. I just did step one, and after ninety days, I went out speaking. I thought that was enough. I had a lot of secrets I didn't want to talk about. I really thought I would never drink again. I see now I was only dry during this period.

I moved back to the Bronx in 1989 and I still went to meetings . I had a home group. I lived at the Desperados' clubhouse. It was near Arthur Avenue by 188th Street. I left the Desperados to prospect for the Hell's Angels. I haven't had a drink in six years, but I was into violence. I prospected for eighteen months and became a Hell's Angel on July 31, 1993. I made it; I had hit the big time. I was a big shot in my mind. But the pride comes before the fall. By this time, I really didn't go to too many 12 step meetings; I went once in a while. I was too busy being a tough guy in the Hell's Angels. I wasn't drinking and I thought I was all right. I was doing what I wanted to do.

Things began to go wrong in my life in 1995. I went to Paterson on my motorcycle and was putting up flyers in some bars about a party we were going to have for Cochise, who was a Hell's Angel. I was warned by some of my brothers that there might be trouble because we knew the Pagans hung out at these bars. I went ahead and did it anyway. When I left the bar, I realized a car was following me; I tried to get away. They crushed me while I was riding my motorcycle into a parked car very hard and very fast. I was left for dead, but somehow I survived. I was hurt very badly and taken to the hospital, where I stayed for three days. I went back to the clubhouse where I lived on Third Street in Manhattan. Some of my brothers were pissed at me because of what happened. Later on in June, I had to have leg surgery. I was waiting to get better because I planned on getting revenge and also shutting up certain brothers who I knew were pissed at me. I went back to work in September and got a job at Newark Airport, doing concrete work. I am in the Laborers' Union. I worked there one week. When I came to work on a Monday, there were two Pagans working there. I knew who they were and they knew me. I said everything was all right. I was kind of surprised to see them, and I didn't know what to do. We had to have passes to work at the airport. There was a lot of extra security because the trial of the sheik that tried to blow up the World Trade Center in 1993 was going on. So I let it go. I didn't think it was a smart move to try to do anything there. When I went back to the clubhouse, I told a few of the brothers about the Pagans at the airport. They turned on me and said I made the club look bad, and if I didn't do something about it I would be kicked out. The next day, I beat up one of the Pagans. I lost my job and had to leave the airport. I got voted out of the Hell's Angels at the next meeting.

My whole world caved in. I was full of fear and I was all alone and hurting. I was angry at them and myself for getting kicked out. I drifted around. But I still wasn't drinking. I don't know why; I was sure set up for it. I was full of resentment and self-pity. I did start to drink again in 1997. Goodbye twelve years and three months of no drinking. I hated myself; I couldn't blame anyone. I drank it. I tried recovery a few times; I was in and out. I got a room in the Bronx and went to meetings up there. I kept drinking off and on, and I was doing some cocaine. I did end up in detox in the Bronx in 1998. It was there that I was told that I had hepatitis C. I took it like a death sentence. I continued to drink and do cocaine. I didn't care. I hated myself.

I got kicked out of my room in the Bronx for drinking. I ended up in a hotel on Route 46 in Jersey. I considered suicide. I got a room in Garfield and I came back to the 12 step program. I went to meetings at the Sahara Club. I knew some of the people there from before. I told them I was coming back. I bounced around and I got a bunch of ninety-day pins. I kept drinking. I kept trying. I wouldn't give up. I had hope. On June 20, 2001, I had my last drink. I knew what I had to do, so I got busy right away. I got a sponsor and I wrote my life story and also wrote my fourth step. I knew I would get drunk again if I didn't. I did something about my tough health battle. I had many side effects from the medicine. It was at this point in my life that I found my higher power. He lives within me. He gave me the hope and the strength to battle this hep-C virus. The viral load test went from more than 200,000 to less than 50. They called it remission. I call it a miracle. I am still fine thirty-one months later. I really cleaned house. I wrote a lot about my recovery and let people read it; It helped me. I went to three meetings a day. I read the Big Book. I wasn't working, because I was sick from the treatments for the hep C virus, so I wrote about my deep, dark secrets. I got rid of the things that haunted me. I prayed to my higher power to give me the strength. I felt deep shame about these things. He gave me the strength and I thanked him for it. I talked about the sexual abuse, how I hated and blamed myself for it. I wrote to my sister and one of my brothers about it. I also talked about how

I let gay men perform oral sex on me for drinking money, mostly on Forty-second Street in the '70s. I had shame and guilt. I hated myself for all of it. I also had sex with some transsexuals, and that did a number on my brain. I feared that I would become a homosexual because of what that man did to me. I did some self-abuse. I was really sick and I hated myself. I was into violence. I got into a lot of fights on Forty-second Street. I told my sponsor about all of these things.

I went on a retreat my first year in recovery. where I met a priest who kept talking about how victims don't heal. You can get better by forgiving and praying for people you hate. I told him my story and let him read some of my stuff. I began to pray for certain people. I wanted to get rid of the hate. I began to pray for that man who stole my innocence. I prayed for health, happiness, and good fortune for him. I have also prayed for my old brothers, the Hell's Angels. I felt resentment because of what happened. I prayed for good things for them. I do pray for my enemies, the Pagans, the Outlaws, and the Bandidos, and the two people in the car who tried to kill me. I have prayed for my father, who died because of his drinking in June 1979. I ask God to be kind to him. He was a sick man. I hope God has mercy on him. I don't pray every day for these people—it is hard praying for your enemies. It is a tough concept to understand. I know this can be done. I was told a story by this priest on the retreat about two women who survived the Nazi concentration camps. They met 45 years later and talked about the war. One mentioned how one of the Nazi guard's got caught and how happy she was because she hated them. The other one said to her I forgave them . The first women couldn't understand how she could forgive. The other women stated "you are still there prisoner forty five years later and I'm not."So I said to myself if she could forgive them I can forgive people too

I am going to therapy now. I have gone three times so far. I hope it will help me. I go there mostly for the sexual abuse issues. I want to put it behind me. I have to learn to live in the moment. I am trying to move on with my life. I committed a lot of crimes in my old life. I don't do those things anymore. They weren't very good for me or anyone else. I can be a better person. I have to practice these things daily. The twelve steps teach me to accept the things I can't change, and to work on the things I can change.

I have been going to a 12 step meeting for survivors of alcoholic families on Sundays for six months. It seems to help. After all, I was affected by alcoholism in my family before I became an alcoholic. I believe my higher power wants me to attend all these kinds of meetings. I do need the extra help. I have my dignity and self-respect back.

Life is a journey. My recovery is the most important thing in my life today. I have to walk the walk. Lip service is for free. I will continue to do the work. I need to grow up; I still have childish behaviors. I work really hard. I have to learn how to relax; the joy of living is the theme of the twelfth step. I have to practice this.

Anyway, I have done a lot of wrongs in this life, but I did some things right too. I have made foolish decisions. I have made honest mistakes. What am I trying to say? I am human—no more, no less than anyone else. I am making progress. I need to understand singleness of purpose; stick to the recovery principles; practice these principles in my life. I have faith and I do the work. I have started therapy and I go to two other meetings for other issues. I believe this is what my higher power wants. He is the healer. Love is the greatest healer of all time. We can overcome anything. God and working a 12 step program can fix broken people like me. They take us out of the gutter and put us back on our feet. I am so very grateful for all of the miracles, my own and others'. recovery is full of miracles. A grateful alcoholic won't drink today. I am grateful to be sober forty-four months, and I am grateful to be in remission from hepatitis C for thirty-three months. As I have said, my recovery program comes first. There is no compromise about this. I am getting better. We can't change our past, yet we can be better people today one day at a time.

I don't always know what I want out of life. I do have peace and inner strength. I have my hopes and my dreams. Of course, life has a way of crushing my dreams. What is it all about anyway? I had my fifteen minutes of fame when I was a Hell's Angel. I was in the newspaper a few times. I am at a crossroad. Soon I will be moving. I go to a lot of meetings. I believe in giving back. You get out of recovery what you put into it. I am still a loner but I am not alone. I have my higher power who lives within. Hope lives right there. It is down deep inside. I guess it is my soul. I have hope in my life. I found reasons to keep on living. I am a hepatitis C survivor. I am living with it. I am not letting negative emotions rule my life. I still have fears. I have fear of hepatitis C coming back. I don't want to have to go on that treatment. It was very tough. Interferon and Ribaviran are the two drugs I took. I had to take three shots a week of interferon. I did more than 100 shots. I told myself that three times a week I had 3 million tiny little marines put into my body to fight the virus; thank God for the marines. We won the war. What a miracle. I am still fine thirty-three months later. I can never say how grateful I really am. I must continue to work on myself. My higher power is good to me. He gives me what I need daily. Thank God for the 12 steps and second chances.

I don't have a girlfriend in my life, mostly because I don't try. I haven't had a girlfriend since 1995. Anyway, I have to let the emotional scars of the sexual abuse heal. I cannot go on living in denial. Today I have many female friends slowly the healing process has begun. I have to face the facts about my life. I am growing up. I became a recluse after I got kicked out of the Hell's Angels. I write to them, and I did look into getting a second chance. I know they are coming to Jersey. I had hoped I would get a second chance.

It didn't turn out that way. Anyway, my expectations caused me pain.

And so, life is a journey. Things come and go. People come and go. Life will go on, with you or without you. I had to start over many times. I lost everything when I got kicked out of the Hell's Angels. I was sleeping in the back of a van. I was homeless and I wasn't drinking. I have done violent things to people and violent things have been done to me. I was almost murdered in 1995. There has been a lot of loss. Anyway, it all had to happen just the way it did because I had to hit a new bottom. The new bottom was when I considered suicide on that last drunk.

Today I am somebody. I am decent. I am kind and loving. I have made mistakes in the past and I will make mistakes in the future. Life is hard. So what—that's no excuse to drink. It doesn't solve problems. Once an alcoholic, always an alcoholic. At this moment, I am on unemployment. I have put my name on the out-of-work list at the Union Hall. What is different is that I have a sponsor and I have done the twelve steps to the best of my ability. I will continue to go over them, growing pains in sobriety, it is an inside journey. I have to clean the garbage out of my life so the good can come in. It is character building. I've got a good support crew. It isn't that big, but it works. I give back to the programs . To me, gratitude is an action. I am responsible for my own recovery. I can't change the past, but I can learn from it. I hurt a lot of people with my crimes and my violence and also with my mouth. I don't commit crimes today, and sometimes I say things I wish I didn't say, but I am getting better.

So where do I go from here? I've got a new place to live. I will still go to meetings in the club. I have been going to the doctor's a lot. I get frustrated. I have been sick almost forty-four months, but it is all right because I have learned to accept it. I take four kinds of medicine. I am very grateful for my good results with the hepatitis C virus. It is very hard to let go of the past.

One of the Hell's Angels got killed in Philly a few weeks ago. They are at war with the Pagans. It brought back memories of when I was almost murdered. I am going on with my life. I am a survivor. I will be forty-eight years old in June. I also will be sober four years in June. I didn't have a lot in life. I don't have a wife or a girlfriend, kids or a home. I believe my sobriety is my success. We can overcome some very steep odds. I am going on a retreat in March to work on childhood issues. It is my first one with that fellowship. I am looking forward to it. I am so very grateful for all the miracles in my life. They used to call me Killer Kane. Today, I am just Richard Kane.

June 2003

My family life at home was all about clean beds made military style, everything had to be put away. Everything had to look good; it was a house of furniture. All the feelings were under the rug. Fear ruled the house. The hurt and pain and the silence were constant. Don't upset the old man or I knew what would happen a beating. Even when they didn't, I always felt like a beating was coming. Love was an unspoken word, rarely heard and seldom felt. Rage and anger were always present. Being put down for not living up to somebody else's expectations was a pretty regular thing. I went to other people's houses as a kid; rarely did they come to mine. At my home, the tension was always there. It was my family, the only one I knew; I had very little self-esteem. As I got older, I became angry and I started to act out on my anger. I hated my family for the façade of being normal; there was very little there. When we moved from the Bronx to Bergen Field, nothing changed; it was still the same crazy family. The old man was all right if you stayed out of his way and didn't bother him. He had no interest in what any of us did. He never gave any compliments. I never heard him say *I love you* to anybody; he always looked angry. I never saw my mom and dad show any affection for one another. My father liked drinking and he hung in the bars. He even had a bar in the basement at our home in Bergen Field. I felt I was always being put down. It seemed like I could never do anything right, so why bother? I learned some lessons such as if I didn't move or make any noise during the beating, then it would end much sooner. I don't know which was worse, the beatings or the put-downs. They both hurt in more ways than one; they hurt me right down to my soul. I felt worthless after the beatings. Feelings weren't talked about; I wasn't supposed to have any. I was always told how I should feel. Every summer, up to about the age of twelve, My younger brother Tom and I would be sent to our grandmother's, one week for each of us, but not at the same time. It was a reprieve from the madness. I always had a good time with my grandparents; we went for walks down by Main Street in Flushing. We played cards, we talked, I ate well. I felt they really cared about me. We never talked about my father's drinking or the other stuff. It was great while it lasted. It ended and then I went home. It was the same old thing: the beatings, no one being around when I wanted somebody to talk to. It seemed nobody cared. Once in a while, something good would happen. It didn't last. I never felt safe where we lived; it was better not to be around. I never slept well. Since we weren't allowed to cry, I rarely did; sometimes I would cry into my pillow so no one would hear it. We used to go to church in the Bronx and Bergen Field on Sunday. My father never came to church; he never went to anything for anybody. We never took vacations. I learned how to hide a lot of things, mostly my feelings. Don't rock the boat or the old man will give you a beating. I am trying to understand what happened to me, and where I came from. As I write this, I am sober a little more than two years. I am doing this because I believe it will help me. I have to see what I learned and what I didn't learn. I am not trying to blame my family. I never learned how to get close to people. I don't even know who I am. Closeness was not a family trait. I felt like people didn't want me around. I also felt alone. I am trying to get down to causes and conditions, as the Big Book says. I know it is going to be painful; we can deal with it together. Richard Kane never grew up. I never felt secure in the world. I was full of fear. I had to learn how to survive. I learned how to be one way with some people and another way with other people. Don't let anybody get inside, so they can't hurt you. I was very self-protective- Because I didn't want to be hurt. I didn't trust my family or other people; I had a fear of all people. I tried not to depend on anyone, and I tried to be self-reliant. It didn't work. I messed up my own life because I wanted to run the show. When I was a kid, my father's drinking caused a lot of problems to the family. I couldn't talk about this stuff, so I never did. I learned to be silent. I lied so much, I started to believe that it was the truth. Sometimes I got blamed for something I didn't do. It didn't matter; I got the beating anyway. I always felt like I was doing something wrong, even when I wasn't. Funny things happen in life, like growing up. Before I knew it, I was a man. I couldn't tell anybody that I was really a scared little kid. . I hid it well. I covered up my fear with drinking and anger. Act tough and nobody will bother me . People are afraid ofme ; it keeps them at bay. Fear is a weapon. It will make me fight harder. I always tried not to depend on people. People didn't want me around because of my drinking and the violence. As I got older, the family got rid of me . I ended up in the gutter. I used to sleep in the parks in Bergen Field, in the monkey barrel.

Anyway, back to the family. As I said, my father's favorite room was the basement. He had his bar and his TV down there. He never ate with the family. I didn't feel comfortable around my father. He could be harsh with his punishments. I remember getting sent to bed with no supper; I remember getting sent to bed after a beating; I remember getting up in the morning with dry blood on my pillow from my head. I learned about terror and fear very young. This was all part of my childhood; it happened a long time ago. Yet I remember it like it happened yesterday. I wonder why things happened the way they did. There is no answer. Don't ask too many questions; it will just bring more pain. I had to learn to live with it; thats how I survived.. I also learned to make believe none of it ever happened. None of these things ever worked because I knew what the truth was. As a child, I never felt special. I only knew great pain. I got beaten and I saw other family members get beaten. When you are small, you are helpless to stop it. You learn to take it. I put the beating out of my mind until it ended. I had nowhere to go to talk about these things. I had to get use to living this way and sometimes I believed I deserved it. No child should be beaten and treated like that. I asked myself why. Again there is no answer My father has his problems; he was a drunk, he was angry a lot, he was in the marines and he fought in World War II. I never did get to know my father; we never talked. I tried to avoid him. I was afraid of him. I stayed out of his way. I knew he couldn't beat me if I wasn't around. I am trying to learn about myself. I need to get some understanding. That is why I am writing about these things. I also had sexual abuse. I was under ten when it happened. It was a stranger. It happened in the Bronx. It only happened once. I never told anyone about this for about forty years. Fear played such a big part in my life, I learned. If I looked good, nobody really noticed that I was messed up inside. . We never talked in my family. We all kept secrets. You know silence is golden. Didn't Frankie

Valli sing that in his song? When I look back at my life, it seems like it was all a bad joke. I learned to laugh. Never cry, because that would get me a beating. I paid the price for not learning how to deal with my problems . I believe .I have to learn how to deal with the past and put it behind me. The funny thing is, everything I hated about them, I became. I hated my father's drinking as a kid. When I got older, I became a drunk. Ihated his violence; I became violent when I got older. I could be cruel sometimes. So broken homes produce broken children who later on in life become broken people. The good news is that God and 12 step programs can fix a broken person like me. I am willing to do the work to become a better person. I am putting it on paper for other people to read it. It will help me in the healing process. It breaks down the denial. No one said it was going to be easy. I believe I am going to get better because I am taking action. The search is inward. I need all the help I can get. It is one hell of a journey. It isn't always so pleasant. God knows me better than I know myself. I trust my higher power. I want to get better. The obstacles are many. They are being dealt with, one at a time and slowly. I still hold on to some of my old self. It is hard to change. The fears are still there. The isolation is a part of the fear of people. I feel safe when I am alone. I do know great loneliness. I have a hard time breaking these patterns. I have done them for so long. I have found courage so I can change and become a better person. Love is the greatest healing power in the world. God's love heals. I still have a problem with human love. I trust God and the program . I don't trust every person in the program . I know it is fear. I have to keep cleaning house. The change has to happen inside. I do have meaning to my life today thanks to recovery and my higher power. I have gone through the twelve steps. Clearing away the past has to be done so I can live better today. I have another illness. I have hepatitis C. There is no cure for it. It is treatable and beatable. I believe in miracles. I am in remission twenty-eight months. We can overcome so much together. Letting go of the past is hard. I have my memories of my family, my crimes, the years I spent in jail, the rehab, the motorcycle clubs, the Desperadoes and the Hell's Angels, the violence, and the sexual abuse. Life can be cruel. Today I am responsible for my own life. I can start a new life in recovery by practicing the principles of love, hope, and forgiveness. I am becoming more tolerant. I am learning patience. I am also learning about kindness, so today I think I am doing pretty good. I am very grateful for all the chances I have been given .

January 2007

I look back so I can learn. I realize that pain has its good side. The pain of how I was living brought me back to the program . I try to learn how to live with myself. I accept my imperfection. I am human. I can accept my wounded ness. It started in my family. Things happened . I got a lot of physical beatings. I felt out of place; I was always uneasy. I liked to run away. I would run all around the West Bronx. I liked to go down by the Harlem River. I was always in trouble. It seemed like I couldn't do anything right, so why try? I remember when that man got me on the tracks. He was friendly at first, until he was behind me. My pants were down. I didn't know what he was doing. I was only seven. It hurt and I wanted him to stop. The train came and people got off. He held my mouth and told me to shut up. No one saw it. It was dark. He finished and he let me go. I ran away. I remember the blackout in 1964. I was out on 181ˢᵗ Street in Washington Heights. I was seven. I was shoplifting in Woolworths. I came home late and for once, my father was there. He was mad at me for being out. I got a beating. I went to bed; we had bunk beds. I was on the top. I knew all the bars on Ogden Avenue. I have been in all of them, looking for my father. It is funny how in the bars, every person I met was a friend of my father's, They were always drinking. The bars were always dark. They had a color TV; we had black and white. I remember moving to Bergen Field, New Jersey, a new world. People had lawns. I had to cut the grass and rake the leaves. The kids didn't play in the street like we did in the city. I had to get used to that. I liked to play sports. I did pretty well. I learned how to play all the sports on my own and from other kids. I watched baseball and football on TV and tried to be like the pros. When I began to drink at eleven, I lost all interest in sports, I mean playing. I watched sports however on TV and I drank whenever I watched a game. Life goes by very fast. I went away for my first time at fifteen. I got arrested a bunch of times. I was charged with sixteen burglaries in a bunch of towns, and for stealing a car. I laughed about all of it. I didn't care what they did to me. I didn't know how to talk to people. I didn't get along with people. I was angry and I got in a lot of fights. I carried the burdens of my sexual abuse and the beatings by myself. I hated myself and I thought I was worthless. I never tried to change. People did try to help. The courts sent me to a couple of rehabilitation centers . .

I was honest about some things. I always drank again anytime I got out of jail or the hospital or the detox center or one of the many rehabs; I was a loser. My journey went on. I stopped drinking for more than twelve years. I went back to the bottle in 1997. When the bottle was empty, so was I. I am sober since June 20, 2001. I am very active in the meetings. I also attend other twelve-step groups. When I became a teenager, I looked up to men of violence. I remember seeing motorcycle gangs in the '70s in Bergen Field, "the Huns" they were called. I wanted to be like that. Of course, everyone knew of the Hell's Angels. My father was a marine. I tried to get into the army; I took the tests, but I was denied because of my record. I did state time for a burglary. It was after the Vietnam War, probably 1979 or 1980. Well, anyway, I remember when I got ten months on Rikers Island in New York. I got into a fight in the

Port Authority on Forty-second St. I was drunk and in a blackout. I gave one of the cops a black eye and I got a beating by the cops. I was still on parole in Jersey, so we made a deal. I pled guilty and got ten months; no big deal. I was used to that kind of life. I looked up to the West Side mob, the Irish. I met some of them in Rikers. I wanted to hook up with them but it never happened. I got out, I got drunk; what else is new? I realize now that I was looking to fit in anywhere I could. I had no self-esteem and I was trying to get it from others. I see clearly how messed up I really was. Booze seemed to take all the pain away. I was a broken person who was lost. I just wanted to fit in; I wanted to feel love. I wanted somebody to tell me I was all right. I had a lot of shame hidden deep inside. I didn't know how to get rid of this stuff—the inner conflict, the voices in my head telling me I was no good, I was stupid, I was ugly. I felt worthless and I couldn't forgive all of the things that happened. I blamed myself for the sexual abuse. I would never talk about it; it was well over forty years before I began to do something about it. I covered up my bad feelings and low self-worth with working out, being a tough guy, not caring. I became a Desperado. That was my first motorcycle club. I wore the club colors; it made me feel important and tough. My ego got a big boost when I became a Hell's Angel in 1993. This is my story of trying to find my place in life. It is a story of being wounded, being broken, and almost getting murdered. It is the story of finding a reason to live and finding good in myself. It is about moving toward wholeness and acceptance. I accept all the parts of my life; they make me who I am. I am all right.

I am grateful to be sober for more than six years. I am a sexual abuse survivor. I go to a group for that. I also go to therapy. I go to meetings to understand and deal with my alcholic home life. All of this stuff helps me to face myself. I can't hide the past or deny that it happened. I try to face my demons one demon at a time. I can see that since I had no real identity, I would look to gangs or causes to fulfill that for me. I did support the IRA and their fight for Irish freedom. My mother's side of the family is from Ireland. I read all the books about the IRA. I listened to all the rebel music; I even joined Irish Northern Aid. I marched for Joe Doherty in Manhattan at MCC. I was looking for another outlet for my anger. I remember when the ten hunger strikers died. I hated Margaret Thatcher and I wished she was dead. I really liked it when the IRA blew up stuff and killed English soldiers; my views about that have changed since 9/11, and I am glad that they have the peace process in Ireland. I must learn to live with myself. I turn my life over to my higher power, my past, my present, and my future. I do intend to stay sober for the rest of my life, one day at a time. I believe in myself. My higher power is always with me. I ask for guidance. Things confuse me. I am not afraid to make mistakes. I have learned that I am not a mistake. I try to grow daily. I take my lumps like everybody else. I did take some new lumps this year. My girlfriend left me in January; it was very painful for around five to six months because she wouldn't tell me why she left. I am all right with it now I hardly think about her because it isn't so important for me to find out she cannot talk to me; this is her problem. I did learn that I can fall in love, give and get love, and accept rejection. I got hurt but I didn't get broken. I was not romantic. Most of my life I had very low self-esteem and wouldn't even try to be with women. I have had four girlfriends and I am fifty. You can see that I haven't been with that many women. today I am comfortable with who I am. I did have some sexual problems but I don't today. My sexuality is good and God-given and it is a gift. I am not seeing anyone at this time. I did try for a few months with a new woman. I still have strong feelings for her. I am not romantic with her. I do talk to her and see her. I am all right with or without a woman in my life but I would like to have a meaningful relationship one day.

February 22, 2008

Sobriety is the most important thing in my life. I may believe my job or my home life comes first, but I must remember, if I don't get sober and stay sober, chances are I won't have a job, a family, sanity, or even life itself. If I am convinced that everything in my life depends on my sobriety, I have a better chance of getting sober and staying sober. If I put other things first, I am only hurting my chances. Lots of meetings, lots of chances; some meetings, some chances; no meetings, no chances. Don't drink; go to meetings; read the Big Book; do the work; grow up; change; stay sober.

Richard Kane
sober date June 20, 2001

May 11   Affirmations (1)   Richard Kane

Sober date June 20, 2001

Sobriety is the most important thing in my life. I honor and respect my body. I am learning to take good care of myself. My relationships are mirrors that show me myself. I am now an open channel for creative energy. God is showing me the way. I am now being guided to the perfect solution to this problem. I love myself and I naturally attract loving relationships. I now feel deep inner peace and serenity. I am glad I was born, and I love being alive. I love myself as I am. I give thanks now for all the good that I have and all the good to come. Every day I am growing healthier and more attractive. I now let go of all guilt, fears, resentment disappointments, and grudges, I am free and clear. God is the strength in which I trust. Everyone wants the kind of love I have to offer. Love waits on welcome, not on time. Gratitude goes hand in hand with love. To forgive is to heal. To love myself is to heal myself. I teach only love, for that is what I am. Listen silently and learn the truth of what I really want. I am now releasing my past. The light within me is creating miracles in my body. I am now creating my life exactly as I want it.

Dec 2007

Life is a journey and there are lessons to be learned. I continue to try to grow up. I am dealing with all my issues. I go to all kinds of twelve-step meetings. I am in recovery for everything. I go to therapy once a week. Rich Kane, the beaten, battered, abused street kid from the Bronx, is a survivor.. I don't run away from my problems. I am not afraid of life or people. My journey through life has taken many twists and turns, from growing up on 170th Street and Merriam Avenue in the Bronx. I took many physical beatings as a youth. I adjusted to that. I learned to hide my feelings. I also learned how to put my mind out of body as a kid so I could take blows and not move or cry or show any emotion. Because of this The beatings would end sooner, but there was always another one. I knew great fear as a kid. I didn't feel safe around my father; I thought he hated me. I used to run all around as a kid. I would go all over the city, down by the Harlem River, across to Washington Heights on the High Bridge. Sometimes we would sneak into the pool in High Bridge Park. Sometimes we would swim in the Harlem River. I used to shoplift on 181st Street in Washington Heights. I would also shoplift on Fordham

Road. I could go all around New York on the subway; we would sneak on them, me and the others kids from the High Bridge neighborhood, right near Yankee Stadium. My grandmother lived close to Yankee Stadium. I liked Yankee Stadium. It was on River Road, right by the train on 161st Street. I went to Sacred Heart Catholic School on Nelson Avenue. I didn't do very well in school. I was too hyper and I was mirror-minded; I wrote backwards. I am left handed. I couldn't sit still; I still have that problem. Even though I got a lot of beatings from my father, I still love him and I forgive him.

We left the Bronx in 1967 when I was ten. I didn't want to leave. We came to Jersey and things remained the same. I stuffed my feelings all my life. I found booze when I was eleven or twelve. I loved it; it made me feel good. It helped me to forget all the pain. Booze was my best friend. I was really messed up inside. I couldn't tell people about these things. I hated myself and I blamed myself for so many things. I started to get in a lot of trouble. I was arrested many times. I really believed I was evil; there was something wrong with me. I thought I was ugly. I drank all my feelings away. I had no plans or goals in life.

I just got into a lot of trouble and I would get sent away a lot. I thought everybody hated me. I didn't think people wanted me around. Life happened so fast; before I knew it, I was an adult. I knew about jails, the hospitals, all of those places that booze and my actions took me to. What can I say? I am fifty; I am sober six and a half years; I am in remission from hepatitis C for more than five years. I am grateful to be sober and free. I am somebody; I am a decent, kind, caring, loving human being. I have value. I try to help others. My life is centered on living the twelve steps, having a higher power, and trying to do the right thing. I can look back at my life to see how many times my higher power God saved me. I fell off the store roof in the Bronx one story high.when I was under ten. I survived that. Even when that man sexually abused me, he could have killed me. My higher power was there. I have a lot of scars. I have had over eleven operations., some due to my 5 or 6 bike accidents. I've been in a lot of fights. I almost got murdered. My higher power kept me alive for some reason. I will try to serve that purpose. I made a mess of my life; I accept that. I can't fix it. God and recovery can and they have. I am grateful. I am not afraid of the future. He is with me, He will guide me, He will see me through.

I am going to a lot meetings. I am not working; I am on unemployment. My name is on the out-of-work list down at the union hall.

March 26, 2008

I cannot change anything until I own it as my own. I take responsibility for my feelings today. I own my past, I own my fear and sadness. I mourn the loss of my childhood. I realize I didn't get the things I needed as a child. I don't blame, I accept what happened. I turn the past over to my higher power. He makes something good out of the ruins of my life.

I felt shame; I felt lonely. I was full of fear; I was hurt; I felt powerless. I was afraid of my father and I didn't trust my mother. I got a lot of physical beatings. It was a cold harsh home. It was always lonely, with no noise. There were no feelings in the home, no love or encouragement. I felt like a burden. I felt I wasn't wanted. Was it true? I don't know. It was crazy; it was an insane place to live. I didn't have feelings. I only knew anger. When I got older, I thought it empowered me. I had a lot of violence in my life. I was violent to others. I became a drunk as a teenager. I hid all my feelings, the deep shame, the guilt, the blame. I always thought I was doing wrong, even when I wasn't. I was unsure of myself. I hid it all by being cocky and tough. I didn't know how to get along with people. I always felt people were out to hurt me. Was it true? I doubt it. I had no plans or goals as a teenager. I just got in a lot of trouble; that was a big part of my image. I had trouble staying still. I was always on the go. Wherever I was, I didn't want to be there. So I went somewhere else. I didn't want to be there either. I was on the run. I couldn't hide from myself. I had to stop one day and look. I didn't like what I had seen, so what was I going to do about it? I had to change. I went slowly. I worked on my attitude. I worked on how I felt about myself. I had to get rid of old negative beliefs. I let my higher power replace them with new positive beliefs. I will continue to grow. I am sober since June 20, 2001. I am very grateful. I am looking forward to a new day in the future when I can relax and not work as hard on my recovery. I hope to someday stop going to therapy. I do want to learn to live in the now. I still drift into the past. I am a survivor. I am growing. It is slow sometimes. I do slide back. I keep on going ahead. I have faith in my higher power. I need to learn to let go and let God. Old habits die hard. I have to practice new ways of doing things. I am working on being free of my past. Only my higher power can do this. I can live better in the day as long as He is in control. All things are possible with God. I can learn how to respond to life. God's love can heal all my wounds and scars. Can I allow the spirit of God to do this for me? It takes a lot of work to allow God to heal me I sometimes get in the way. I realize that I paid a price for not dealing with my problems. I ran and hid in a bottle of booze. I was numb and in a fog. I didn't care; the price I paid for this wasn't the one on the bottle. I have meaning in my life. Can I learn to live for my higher power? Will I let my higher power empower me? Will I allow my will to be transformed for the highest good? These are not easy things to do. I practice this stuff; it is only God's grace that I am sober. I must continue to grow. I must face my problems, look at them, and deal with them. It is necessary for me to be in the solution. I gave my power to a bottle. I thought it was doing something for me. I got that glow from booze, but it was a false glow.

I now have a glow from being in 12 step recovery and I thank God for that. . My old life was a dead life; it was the walking dead, a life of illusion and make-believe, a fantasy world. Can I embrace reality? Can I live in the now? Will I allow the Holy Spirit to transform me? I am in recovery. I participate in my recovery. The truth will set me free. I keep it simple. Booze is not the answer to any of my problems. I try to live in the solution. I want to live in the sunlight of the spirit. I have a small relationship with my higher power. I am growing; the spirit is guiding me. I still have free will. I am human. I will fall short. I can make a mistake; I am not a mistake. I can fail; I am not a failure. I am a success because I am sober. Sobriety is a gift. Will I cherish it? Am I grateful to have it? My actions will show that I am. I go to many kinds of meetings; I also go to therapy. I need all the help I can get. I believe it is working. I am getting better. I have learned that I don't have to carry the false guilt and shame from my childhood sexual abuse; I did that to myself. I sentenced myself to that false pain for more than forty years. That person stole my innocence; he committed a crime against me. I am no longer a victim. I have brought it into the light to be healed; it is being healed slowly. I no longer blame myself. It is just something that happened because I was the one who was there. It was a stranger. I have forgiven this person, although I haven't forgotten it. I must work on forgiveness as much as I can on a daily basis. It comes slowly and in degrees. I am not owned by my past. I can live in the day; I am free of this burden.

March 1 2008

I remember as a child the places I would go in my mind to escape the pain. I would have to stand without moving and show no emotion while I was getting beaten. I could not cry; I wasn't allowed. I knew if I didn't, the beatings would end sooner. It's funny how those lessons stayed with me. My family was my first teachers I learned to look but not really see. I knew better than to say anything. Everybody made believe everything was all right; I learned to put on the face, the façade. Everything was clean and neat; it hid the chaos and the terror that lurked just beneath the surface. All the feelings were hidden under the rug. I learned very young not to be around. I learned how to lie; I learned how to make believe everything was all right. It was my family; it was all I had. The alcoholic home is full of distortions. I pretended , I ignored I stayed away, I made believe, I didn't hear the arguments. I knew about the cold, harsh, critical look. I knew violence could come at any moment when my father was home. Things could go from bad to worse in a heartbeat. I learned to hide all my feelings. I did not trust my father or my mother. I couldn't really talk to them. If I did, I always felt like I was on trial. It is sad to realize and accept that this is the reality of my family life. I realize that I am responsible today for getting better and doing the work. I have to give myself the things I didn't get as a child. I am in the process of doing this. My higher power loves me and is with me and guides me. I ran my whole life. I found the bottle; it took away the pain. I wanted to stay drunk all the time. I am very grateful to be sober. I thank my higher power for the gift of sobriety. I accept my whole life. I ask God to help me to turn it over. I give God my past, my present, and my future. I have made peace as much as I can with my past. I do forgive all of the people who harmed me. I am doing all right. I do intend on staying sober for the rest of my life, one day at a time. Drinking is not the answer to any of my problems. I go to a lot of meetings. I attend a meeting for sexual abuse survivors. I have learned to live with it. I don't blame myself. I was an innocent child. I was seven when it happened. I have prayed to God to forgive this person. He was a stranger. I will continue to go to all of my 12 step meetings , therapy, group therapy, and sexual abuse survivors meeting. I pray for the strength to stay on this path. I haven't had a drink since June 20, 2001. I thank God for all of the miracles in my life.

April 2008

To Dad: These are the things I never got to ask you. Did you love me? You never said it. I never did get to know you. You were never around. Drinking in the bar seemed more important. I remember the Bronx and looking in all the bars on Ogden Avenue. It really isn't a very nice place for a little boy. How come you never took the time to talk to me? Why did you beat me so often? Why did you make me march? Couldn't you see the terror in my eyes? Was that what you wanted? Do you remember when I had to make the bed so perfect? I remember when you came into the room with the white glove. You always found dust; of course there was a beating. I remember when we moved from the Bronx to Jersey. I liked sports. I got in the Little League in Bergen Field, and played for the VFW. We only won five games out of twenty. I was a starter. I played right field. I didn't make the all-stars. I did pretty well. I got a decent amount of hits. Why didn't you ever come to watch me play? When I got older, I played in the Pony League; I played first base. I did all right. You never came to watch. Didn't you care about me? Do you remember when you beat me with the hedge clippers on top of my head? Why couldn't you talk to me?

Why did you always punish so hard? I think you would have killed me that day. Jeanine my sister was there; she cried and asked you to stop, and you did. Couldn't you see the pain you caused? I was your son. Didn't you love me? It always seemed like I could do nothing right. I gave up trying very young. I learned to take a good beating and keep my mouth shut. Why didn't you hang out with me and teach me? You never showed me anything. I always thought you were mad at me. You always looked angry. I was too afraid to ask you anything. I knew you didn't want to be bothered. I was a little boy; I was not a marine or a soldier. I needed you; I needed a father. You weren't there for me or anybody else. I realize your drinking was the reason. I did hate your drinking. As a kid, I said to myself I would never be like that. Who knew I would be a drunk and a troublemaker as a teenager? I started to get in very serious trouble. I was arrested a lot for burglaries. I remember getting drunk with you in Bergen Field. You were out of the house because of the divorce. I was out of the house because I was always in trouble with the law and I was sent away. You know, Dad, I was sexually abused at age seven by a white man on the railroad tracks by the Harlem River. I never went and told you. I was too afraid that you would blame me and beat me.

Was I right? You remember all the times I got hurt when we lived in the Bronx? I fell off the store roof. Remember when I almost cut my finger off? How about when I fell on that plank in the alley and the nail went through my hand? Oh, I could handle pain thanks to you.

Well, Dad, I know you are dead since June 9, 1979. Your drinking shut down your liver at age fifty-six. Dad, I forgive you. You were sick; you never got help and you couldn't do your best. Sick people can't. Booze took your life. I want to let you know that I am sober and in recovery. I haven't had a drink since June 20, 2001. Your other son Harold, my older brother, is sober. I think he is sober fourteen years. You realize you taught me not to cry as a kid. There were a lot of tears that were never shown. They stayed on the inside. Our house was full of pain, sadness, silence, fear, and terror. I have a good life today, thanks to all of my recovery groups, group therapy, and a group I go to for sexual abuse survivors. I just want to let you know I am all right. I still think about you. I don't hate you anymore. I forgive you and I love you. I pray that God forgave you too.

Richard

May 1, 2005

To Dad: Did you love me? You didn't seem to have a lot of time for me. I was clumsy; I spilled things. You reacted harshly; you were cruel. You beat me a lot. I was afraid of you. I was afraid to ask you things. You weren't around much. You were silent and you were always angry. You were my father. I needed you. Where was the love? I stayed away from the house. I avoided you as much as I could. You didn't encourage me. You showed no affection. I felt like a burden. Maybe I was a mistake; maybe you didn't want me. I know you are dead a long time. You died on June 9, 1979. I forgive you. It takes two parents to make a family.

To Mom: Why did you compare me to others? I felt you were putting me down. I couldn't measure up to your standards. Why couldn't you accept me? You always tried to change me. You did give some love and encouragement. I know you had it hard; my father was a violent drunk. I don't know why things turned out the way they did. You had to work nights. We had food and we had clothes; I thank you for that. I liked to talk; sometimes I couldn't shut up. I must have been a pain in the ass. I was always getting hurt. You got angry when I got hurt. You took me to the hospital a lot. I would laugh the pain away. I would never cry. Weren't you glad to have me? I am your son. I wasn't always sure if you really wanted me. I had shame as a kid. I was sad a lot. No one was ever around. The place was always clean. There is more to a family than a clean room and food. I am sorry I turned out the way I did. I became a messed-up person. I carry many of the scars of my childhood. I am not blaming. I am responsible for my own life. Today I am sober thanks to God and my recovery meetings.

November 27, 2007

I remember being five or six and getting another beating, who knows for what. Maybe I spilled the milk. The blows are too many to count. I only have ten fingers. I was not allowed to show any emotion. I take my mind to that secret place where I don't feel the pain; it is deep inside. The beating ends; I survived another one. The beatings pile up over the years. Who could count that high? I laugh to myself. I will never cry outwardly. I always felt worthless after a beating; funny how that works. Flashback: I am seven; I am on the tracks by the Harlem River. This man is doing something to me. I don't know what it is. My pants are down to my ankles. He is behind me. The train comes in. People get off. He holds my mouth. He tells me to shut up. I am afraid and I am hurt. I can't get away. He finishes. He lets me go. I run; I don't remember where I went. I doubt I went to the apartment. It is funny how these events stay around in my mind. I used to run away. Sometimes I would go to grandma's on Anderson Avenue in the Bronx. She would play Irish records. Macnarma's Band, Danny Boy. Dear Old Donegal. I liked to run the streets of the West Bronx. We lived in High Bridge. We moved to Jersey when I was ten. I was sad. I didn't want to leave my friends, Rickey and Lonnie Parker (they were black) and the Moore twins, Kevin and Kenneth (they were Irish). I remember Alice Hand and Jodie Clark; her mom owned the candy store on Ogden Avenue in the '60s. It seems like yesterday. We ended up in Bergen Field. I started drinking very young. Trouble followed. I was arrested a lot. I got sent away at fifteen. I stuffed all my feelings for so long. I only knew anger. The alcohol helped bring that out. When you survive the kind of life I had, you don't talk about those things. Moving along, I stopped drinking in April of 1985 for more than twelve years. We know what happens to people who stop going to meetings. I got drunk and had my last drink on June 20, 2001.. I am back inrecovery, this time I got a sponsor. I am doing the work. I wrote my life story. I go on retreats. I started going to other meetings dealing with growing up in a dysfunctional home,. I think I was sober around three years when I started to deal with my childhood. I began to go to a meeting for sexual abuse survivors. I meet Colleen my therapist. I started to see her at her office. In April of 2007 I had some EMDR's(eye movement desensitization reprocessing) done with her. They help. I have begun to attend a group she runs. It is a two-year commitment. I can't look at it that way. I can handle one day at a time, one group at a time. Anyway, I am dealing with my feelings and life in general. I can and have overcome many obstacles.

Richard Kane

December 2007: Although I am Bronx-born, I am Irish American. My mother's side of the family is from Limerick, Ireland. My grandfather is from Clare. I always looked up to the Irish freedom fighters, the IRA. I have never been to Ireland. Anyway, when I was locked up in the county jail, I used to read about the Irish people. I had dreams when I was in jail about joining the French Foreign Legion. I also had dreams about going to Ireland and joining the IRA. I studied Irish history; I knew about 1916, the spirit for freedom, Michael Collins, and all of that. I really respected Bobby Sands and the hunger strikers; ten of them died. I remember when the IRA almost got Thatcher with that bomb. I read a lot of books about the IRA . I remember all the bloodshed on the news, the bombings, the ambushes, and the funerals. I really thought they were doing the right thing. The British had put a lot of people in jail who did nothing wrong, the Guilford Four and the Birmingham Six, to name a few. Internment with no charges or a trial had a lot of people locked up. Of course I am an outsider, since I have never been over there. I realize times have changed and things are going very well in Ireland; the peace process seems to be working. I have changed. Time does that. I am fifty and I have mellowed out with age. I realize that as a youth, I was looking for an outlet for my rage and anger, and this cause was one of many things I chose. I see clearly how I was really full of fear and terror, so I became angry as a way of dealing with my feelings. I thought showing rage and anger made me strong. I used to believe violence was the answer to a lot of problems. How wrong I really was. I have come to find peace within. I still get angry. I am human. I don't go into a rage; I don't use violence like I did in the past. I can say that I try to be a better person. I had to remove all of the obstacles from my life so I can stay sober and feel love. I wanted to be accepted, so I joined gangs. I felt unloved and unwanted as a kid. It never went away until I looked at it in my step work. I realize I am human and I need love, so I have learned to love others and myself. I have learned forgiveness. I don't say it is easy; I do know it is necessary. I am fifty. Life goes very fast. I am sober six and a half years. I go to all kinds of meetings. I need to. As a young kid, I had all kinds of violence done to me. I got many severe beatings from my father. I suffered sexual abuse at age seven. That was surely violence and a crime; my innocence was stolen from me. I go to a meeting for sexual abuse survivors. I don't need anybody's permission in my meetings to take care of myself. I go to another twelve-step program It helps me to deal with my upbringing. I don't blame. I look at it as growing pains. I did know right from wrong. So many times I chose the wrong path—the crimes I did, the people I chose to hang with; gang members and hoodlums. I knew I felt out of place with regular people, even though I got drunk again. I gave up more than twelve years of no drinking. I still gained at lot of knowledge and did a lot of good things in that time. I got in the Laborers Union in 1988. I was sober three years. I am still in. This year has been a growing year. I learned some new lessons. My girlfriend broke up with me in January; I was with her seventeen months. She was only my third girlfriend. I also tried to be with another woman; she broke up with me in September. I was only with her a few months. I am all right about all of this. I have real self-esteem, so I can handle these things. I go to group therapy and I talk about my life. I try to count my blessings. I did three retreats this year. I am in a church choir. We sang at one of the retreats . I try to take my own inventory daily. I still need to grow up in certain areas . I still tend to isolatewhich causes me to live alone. I don't like to show my emotions. I still feel out of place with regular people. A lot of my shame has gone away. I still have some habits that I don't like; I have made progress on many of them. My hope is that one day they will go away.

Richard Kane

2-24-07

Oh my lovely Rose of Clare, you're the sweetest girl I know. You're the queen of all, the roses like the pretty flower that grows. You are the sunshine of my life, so beautiful and fair, and I will always love you, my lovely rose of Clare. I am thinking of Nancy as I'm listening to this song. I think I have lost my rose of Clare. It is an Irish love song. I miss her greatly. I have known her for more than four years. We were friends at first. Since the Sahara Club was in Hackensack, she used to come to the meetings with her son, who was very young. We would talk. She was married. She read all my stuff. She knows my story; she knows everything about me, just like my sponsor. It is painful not being able to say hello. She wants zero contact. I miss hearing her voice, her telling me about her day, her son, and her father. We did a lot of things together. We went to the Bronx. I showed her where I lived, even the railroad tracks where the sexual abuse happened. I have learned that even in separation, love is not diminished; love grows stronger. I am deeply in love with her. I have never had anything like this happen before. I am waiting calmly for us to have a chance to talk. I am not willing to just let things end like this. I think if we talk and communicate, we can work through this. When people love each other, they do that. I don't know this for sure. I am taking other people's word about this. I know in my heart how I feel. I am working on change. I have prayed for the removal of my defects. I am going back to therapy Monday. I haven't really slept in five weeks. A lot of stuff came back up: repressed feelings from childhood, the neglect, and no emotional support. I went and told my mother about the sexual abuse. She never knew. When does this stuff end? Does it ever end? The little marine, the beatings, getting my head shoved through a wall. The drawer smashed over my head, the hedge clipper beating. There are many more; I don't want to remember them. I am sick of these memories; they all happened a long time ago, most of them when I was under ten. I am tired of feelings; I wish I never had any. I have worked very hard to get sober. I am trying to learn. I am still sick. I am getting better. I went out with Nancy for seventeen months. She is only my third girlfriend. She is the first person I ever fell in love with. At times I did the best I could. I showed care and concern. At other times, I isolated and stayed away. Low self-esteem, nightmares, and memories stayed in my head. I am grateful this happened; it made me think. It was a wakeup call. I have more work to do. I want to become the person my higher power wants me to be. I am afraid to go back to therapy. I promised a friend I would go. I don't want to look at this stuff again; I want it to go away. I have been thinking about settling down and having a family. Can I do these things? I don't know. I don't want to be a father to someone like I had as a child. I pray to God to help me. I am not angry with her. I hope to talk with her one day and workthrough our differences. I am not looking to be with anyone else. My heart is still with her. Little Nancy, Little Miss Dynamite is what I called her. I still have the hots for her; she is a ten to me. I really admire and respect her. She is my best friend. I am lonely since she broke up with me. I am waiting for her to say when we can talk. I do have expectations. I can't just put her out of mind. It isn't that easy. I am staying sober. I do see her once in a while. We don't talk; she hardly looks at me. I wonder. I know I hurt her, yet the reason wasn't that great. This all happened for a reason maybe she has unresolved issues that she needs to work on.It takes two to have a relationship. The higher good is working on me to get rid of more emotional stuff from the past. I am starting to sleep. I lost about twenty pounds in a month. I feel good. I haven't been taking care of myself the way I can. I have stopped reading. I don't watch TV; I don't listen to the radio. I just sit. I don't pray as much as I used to. I feel rejected. I have hope in the future. I try to turn it over. The future is God's, not mine. It is hard. I want to control. I want the outcome to be a reunion. I have not run away from this. I am going to face it, and get extra help. I need to do these things for myself. I asked God to give me the strength.

2003

To Sonny Barger

This is Richard "Killer" Kane. I am writing to you because I had a dream that involved you, so here it is. I met you and we talked. I told you how proud I was to have been a Hell's Angel in NYC. I got voted in on July 31, 1993. Blues and I made it together; he is still a member. I talked to you about Guinea; he helped me out when I was a prospect. We did hang in Sturgis in '93. I was a member. Mark from Oakland gave me a nice club ring. I met Sharon. I told you about how I got kicked out. I couldn't understand it. I thought I was a decent member. I had become the secretary after being part of the team that beat the government in the building case. I am still proud that I helped. I have been out since October of '95. I still think about it. It is weird that I had this dream. I never met you. I did write to you in prison. I was a prospect. Chip was my sponsor. A lot has happened since 1995. I was sober when I rode with the club. I began to drink again in 1997. I gave up and I threw away twelve years and three months of sober time. I am proud to say I am sober thirty months. You said you were proud of me for going back tothe program. You said you hoped I would stay sober. I told you about my battle with the hep-C virus. I knew you had cancer and you beat it. I told you about the long treatment, the side effects from the drugs. I am in remission for nineteen months. I call it a miracle. It is always darkest before the dawn. I found new strength. I have never been the same since that happened. I call it the light; it lives inside of me, right next to hope. You said you found the same strength to battle cancer. I am happy for your good results and you were happy for me. I am writing to you to help me heal; it helps me to stay sober. I told you how hurt I was because I got kicked out of the charter. I have written to the city for a couple of years. I had heard that the club was going to have a Jersey charter. I was hopeful that I could get a second chance. I did talk to some members about it. I knew I would have to wait to find out what the city would say. I was told I wouldn't be welcomed; it hurt. I have to continue to stay sober. I can't change the past or people. You said I would have to move on with my life, that I should rely on my newfound strength. You also said don't give up hope; nothing is impossible. Well, I thanked you for your time, we hugged, and I said, "I am still red and white in my heart and I will continue to stay sober one day at a time, and who knows? Maybe someday being back in the club can happen." Oh yeah, I have learned a lot in recovery. I take responsibility for my life. We all make mistakes. I am only human. I try to be a better person each day. I can't change the past, although I wish some of it never happened. I had to forgive others and myself so I can move on with my life. I do have to stay sober and this is part of it. Take care of yourself; you have been in the club since 1957; that is the year I was born. With love and respect.

March 22, 2005

I just got back from a retreat; it was a tough weekend. A lot of feelings came back. We did have some laughs and we had some fun. There was a lot of work to do. I came from an alcoholic home; my father was the drunk. I am looking at the family roles all of us played. My older brother Harold was the family hero. He was very smart; my father hated him. He stabbed him one time. He became a drug addict. He is sober twelve years. My sister is older than me. She had no childhood. She had to do everything. She took care of me; she would iron my shirts for Sacred Heart Catholic School on Nelson Avenue in the Bronx. She always looked out for me. My younger brother Tom was the lost child; he was very silent. We used to hang out as kids in the Bronx. And then there was me. I was a hyper kid. I like to talk. I ran all over the streets. I liked to play sports. I liked baseball and football. I played pretty well. I am left-handed. I didn't do very well in school. I liked to run the streets. We would sneak onto the subways and go all over New York City. We were all under ten. A bunch of us kids from the neighborhood hung out together. I liked the Beatles. I also liked the Beatles cartoons. I could sing a little and I could draw. I liked to hang out with Ricky Parker and his brother Lonnie. I also hung out with the Moore twins, Kevin and Kenneth, who lived on Merriam Avenue. I remember the beatings. I also remember the fear. I was afraid of my father. I always had fear that a beating was coming. Even when they didn't happen, the fear was always there. I learned to live with it. I learned to be silent. I made up stories. We lived near Yankee Stadium. Once in a while, I would go to a game. I sat in the bleachers. I liked Mickey Mantle; he was the big star. I saw him hit some long home runs. The football Giants played at Yankee Stadium. I saw one game; I remember Joe Morrison and Homer Jones. I played football. When we moved to Bergen Field, I played Little League baseball for the VFW. There is a lot to think about. I am looking at the inner child picture. I see the stitches, the black eyes, and the scars. I remember going to the hospital a lot. I learned to laugh at pain and never cry; make believe it didn't hurt, and keep my mouth shut. When we moved from the Bronx to Bergen Field, things got worse. I learned to live with the pain. I learned how to take it. By the age of eleven, everything bad that could happen to people happened to me. The violence, the put-downs, the sexual abuse, always being told you weren't good enough. As I got older, I got angry. I thought it helped me to survive. I learned not to care. I become tough; it hides the fear. Fear made me strong for fighting. I had a nickname in Bergen Field; as a teenager, they called me "Krazy Kane." I liked it. I was in trouble all the time. I was arrested for burglaries and stolen cars, also for fighting with the police and shoplifting. I need to write about my feelings from the past, how I was beaten, how I was hurt. I felt no one cared. I had feelings of abandonment. I was sad and sometimes I was lonely. I had many fears. I used to ask myself why. There was no answer; nobody seemed to care. It was better not to be around. I knew I couldn't get a beating if I wasn't around. I became funny; I made jokes out of brutal things that weren't really funny. I was always called stupid. I was put down. I was compared to others. They said I was crazy. I got blamed for things I didn't do. It didn't matter. I got the beatings. I became angry; I became tough. I believed I was evil. I felt I was no good. I gave up trying. I had no one I could talk to about this stuff. I hung in the streets and I found drinking. My parents got divorced when I was in reform school. Once in a while, my mom or my sister or my grandmother would say they loved me. It didn't matter; I felt they were only words. No one knew how I felt. I wouldn't tell them. I didn't think they wanted to know. I never liked myself, and I thought I was ugly. I made up stories so much; I thought they were the truth. I became a sneak, a liar, and a thief. I had a bad temper and I was violent. I had a decent side and I could be kind. In high school, I became a drunk and a loser. I became a jailbird. I can't change the past. So what am I going to do about it now? I am responsible for my own life. I live in the moment and I do the right thing. I have many feelings this morning. I felt good at the retreat. I feel some joy. I went to the dance and I listened to music. I played ball with other people. I went to church and I sang. It made me feel good to watch other people have a good time. Even though my spirit was wounded as a child, it was never fully crushed. My higher power brought me here. I am still a broken person; I am just not as broken. I used to believe broken things couldn't be fixed. I know today that God and working my programs can fix a broken person like me. I have faith and I do the work. I turn the results over to my higher power. I am not blaming my parents. When I got older, I made my own choices. I chose the wrong path. I knew right from wrong. I did a lot of wrong. I became a criminal. My recovery is the most important thing in my life. It is a few days after the retreat. I am in the process of moving. It isn't much. Yet it is better than the streets. When I was a drunk, I lived in the streets. I slept here, there, and everywhere. I was no romantic drunk; I was no Romeo out there. I remember as a teenager how I put myself down. I thought I was ugly. I covered it up with anger and drinking. If people were kind to me, I pushed them away with anger. I had fear of people. It was a sad, lonely life. The blame game kept me down. Drinking in bars put me behind bars many times. When the bottle was empty, so was I. I thought I was a tough guy. I was very arrogant and I thought I could handle anything. I couldn't listen to anybody. I became a slave to alcohol. The bottle ruled my life and it told me what to do and I listened to it. I hated drinking; when I was a kid, I saw what it did to my father. I said to myself as a kid that I would never drink. I look back so I can continue to grow. Times have changed how I look at the past. I am not as angry. I know kids shouldn't be beaten or suffer sexual abuse. I am not alone. I am a survivor. I used to believe my toughness got me through these things. Today I believe my higher power was the one that got me through. Anyway, despite all of that, look at how my life has turned out. I am grateful to be sober forty-five months.

I am in remission from hepatitis C almost three years. I didn't always hate my father. I respected him for being a marine. He did teach me to march and sing the Marine Corps hymn. When I was a kid in the Bronx, I used to go to the VFW on Ogden Avenue with him. He was the post commander. I remember selling poppies with him on 181st Street in Washington Heights. It was in a bar; I think it was the Blarney Stone. Anyway, I think my father had a lot of problems. He died because of his drinking, from liver disease at the age of 56. As a kid, I always wished my father would stop drinking. I wished our family could have been more like some other people's I knew. We never took vacations. We never did much together. There was always tension in the air. The house was always neat. My mom had her flowers. She grew African violets; she won ribbons and she was a state champion. It was her way of dealing with problems. Untreated alcoholism is a killer. I do have some good memories. I went to a Giants football game atYankee Stadium. I think it was 1966. I got in for free, and I sat on the field with the marching band. I loved football and I am a Giants fan. Johnny Curtin took me; he worked at Yankee Stadium. He lived upstairs on the fifth floor,in the same building as us—1406 Merriam Avenue. I remember him drinking beer early in the morning. I had a good time. The Giants lost. I saw Homer Jones score a touchdown. I really liked the hitting in football. Anyway, every summer I would go to my grandmother's for one week. My grandparents moved out of the Bronx and lived in a high rise building on the fourteenth floor in Flushing. I could look right into Shea Stadium from their balcony. They treated me well. We went for walks, we talked, and we played cards. I think they really cared. They were both Irish and they would play Irish records. They would play Macnarma's Band and Galway Bay, all those kinds of songs. I liked those songs; they were happy songs. I always ate well and I would gain weight. When the week was up, I went back home. I was always skinny as a kid. There were six of us in the family. We didn't do much as a family. We had Thanksgiving together. My father's favorite room in the house in Bergen Field was the basement. He had his bar and his TV down there; he never ate with the family. He didn't talk very much. He always looked angry. I tried to stay out of his way. Recovery has taught me that it was all fear. I always seemed to have problems with people. I had very little self-esteem. Self-hatred and anger kept people away. I don't understand life. I was a lost person. I found the bottle; it made me feel good, then it took it all away. When the bottle was empty, so was I. I do have dignity and my own respect now. The bottle took them away. God and all of my work in the program have helped me to get them back. I hope someday to find a companion. I haven't had a girlfriend since 1995. Staying sober is tough work. I have to look at my whole life. So where do I go from here? First things first: I have to stay sober or I lose everything. I have worked very hard to get sober. I have to work even harder to stay sober. God's love is awesome. I am grateful for the miracles in my life. I am sober and I am in remission from hepatitis C.

February 13, 2008

I have come to realize that as far back as I can remember, I felt unloved and unwanted. I received very little love in my childhood. I came from an alcoholic home. There was violence and there was silence. No one seemed to notice that something was wrong. My father liked his whiskey more than anything else. I never got to know him; we never talked. I was very afraid of him, for good reasons. I got tired of the beatings. I see how starved for love and affection I was. I still feel like that at times; I can see how I tried to find peace in the bottle. I wanted to feel like I belonged and someone really cared. To be honest, I didn't feel that way from my family. I was full of fear. I knew terror. What did they want from me? I could never do anything right. After a while, I stopped trying. I just didn't care. I have been hurt. Deep down inside I felt worthless and useless. I remember when I was ten, we moved from the Bronx to New Jersey to the town of Bergen Field. I just got into a lot of trouble at a very young age . I had very little self-esteem. I had a lot of self-hatred. I found the bottle; it was my friend and lover. I couldn't accept myself. I tried to be so tough. I wanted to hide the fear, the terror, and the sexual abuse. I hated my body. I hated the way I looked. I felt ugly and dirty inside. I realize I had no sense of self. I tried gangs—street gangs and motorcycle gangs. I still felt alone. There was a lot of hurt in this life, and I had my fair share. It makes you wonder. The truth is painful. I have gotten backinto recovery. I am sober over six years. I can look back and learn. I see the search. I tried to fit in. I wanted to feel love. I wanted to feel accepted. I didn't have those feelings inside of me. I felt dead. I only felt alive when I was angry. I learned how to fight. I fought a lot in jail. I took pride in the fact that I was a good fighter. I worked out a lot. I still do. My anger isn't so important these days. I am looking deeper at other issues: false pride, being a tough guy, getting esteem from going to jail, being in motorcycle clubs. People respected me because of violence; it was all a cover to hide the zero self-worth that was created by my negative beliefs about myself. I have done the inner child work. I have looked at my childhood so I can learn not to blame. I am responsible for my own life. I have gotten better in a lot of areas. I have learned to feel my feelings and let them go. I stuffed my feelings most of my life. It was a fantasy world. I said my family was normal; what a joke! I am an alcoholic; I am in recovery over six years for a lot of things. I have a higher power in my life. We are getting closer. I have a relationship with this power. I am grateful to the spirit of the universe for sticking with me and giving me another chance. Most people gave up on me. I have been kicked out of my family. I got kicked out of the Hell's Angels. I had two girlfriends break up with me last year. I accept what happened. It was painful. I am not seeing anyone right at this moment. I will try again when the time is right. I have faith. I go to a meeting on Fridays for sexual abuse survivors. I am not a victim. I am empowered by my surrender. I try to turn my life over to my higher power. I do believe in myself. I am all right at this moment. Recovery is slow. It is a lot of back and forth. I keep going on.. I do the work; I leave the results to God. I can see the growth. I had more than six years away from drinking once before; that was in 1991. I was hanging around with the Hell's Angels. I became a prospect in 1991. I went to my recovery meetings once in a while. The reality is, I was on my way back to being a drunk. I did become a Hell's Angel; after eighteen months of prospecting, I was voted in on July 31, 1993. I got kicked out in 1995. Today I go tomy 12 step meetings and I have a sponsor. I still feel lost. I have hope and I take recovery very seriously. I don't have a lot of fun. I have visions that one day I can have a wife and some kids. I feel I can do it now. I can be a good, sober father unlike my own father. I can break the chain of child abuse, sexual abuse, and alcoholism. I have a plan. I believe in the unseen God He is there. He is with me. He helps me with everything I do. I ask for guidance. I need to learn to follow directions. I can make a mistake. I am not a mistake. I am human. I have self-worth. I freely forgive every person who ever did harm to me, and I mean all of it. I also forgive myself for all the harm I did to others and myself. I have come to realize that as I grow older, I see how much I don't know. I want to remain teachable. The spirit of the universe has been really kind and patient with me. I need to learn to be like that with others.

Nov 27, 2007

I look back to learn. I need to get an understanding of my past history. I look at my childhood, not to blame but to process all the wrongs that where done to me . I have to see what I got and what I didn't get. I realize growing up in an alcoholic home gave me distorted thinking. It was not a normal home life. There were beatings and neglect; there was no talking; there was hardly any adult supervision. My sister—a child herself—was supposed to run everything. She got robbed of her childhood; she had to play mom and dad. I was very hyper and I ran the streets of the Bronx. I got injured a lot. I fell of a store roof landing on my head ,I suffered from amnesia. I was playing with the Moore twins. I was under ten when I fell of the roof. It was only one story high. Did you ever wonder why things turned out the way they did? Did you ever ask yourself how come? I became very hard and stopped asking. I became a survivor. You learn to forget. It doesn't work. You learn to ignore; that doesn't work either. Feelings were not shown at all costs. Who knew the true cost? I remember when that man sodomized me at seven years old. That is what they call trauma. I don't know what I called it then. I tried to make believe it never happened. I have dealt with this. I had done an EMDR(eye movement desensitization reprocessing)on this event. I feel my feelings today. I am a little sad this morning. Life goes very quickly. I am not the little Bronx boy; I am not the battered, beaten, bruised, hurt, and scared little child. I am in recovery for everything. I pray for the strength to keep going. There are days I don't want to. I get mentally tired. I get sad. I don't get as angry. I am empowered by my surrender. I have faith. I try to do all the work. I still isolate. I don't really know where I fit in. I know I belong in all of the twelve-step groups I go to. I still feel out of place in society. I can get better and I will trust the process enough to keep trying. The past doesn't own me. I have learned to live with it. I practice forgiveness the payoff gives me peace of mind. I have to believe that the damage from the past can be undone and something worthwhile can come from it. I do have a small relationship with my higher power. I still at times put myself down;and at other times I feel better than other people with prayer and meditation I am striving for balance. I am human; there is a purpose to my life. I have begun to practice giving and receiving love. I am letting down my walls slowly. I don't think people are out to get me. I still get defensive. I pray. I believe prayer changes others and me. I am not sure what my higher power wants .but I am sure he wants me to stay sober to find out. I do have a future. I live in the day. God has a plan for me. I believe most of the plan is about twelve-step recovery and helping others. Can I live up to my end? I try. I had a dream the other day. I dreamed I was in a coffee shop. I fell down. I couldn't breathe; I had died. Some woman I don't know gave me CPR. I came back to life. A stranger breathed the gift of life back into me. She looked Spanish. Then my higher power came to me and whispered in my ear. He said everything was going to be all right and I was to learn how to relax. I then woke up.

Richard Kane

July 15, 2007

I had another EMDR on Friday with Colleen, my therapist. It was very intense and emotional. I almost cried a few times. We did it on the sexual abuse Which occurred in the Bronx on the railroad tracks. HE was a stranger, a man; but he was friendly. He said he would give me fireworks. I was around seven years old. He asked me to take off my pants. I did. He did something; it started to hurt. I wanted him to stop. Then the train came. People got off. He held my mouth and told me to be silent. I did. He finished and he let me go. Colleen said I did nothing wrong. I blamed myself for many years. I was helpless, she said. I wasn't supervised as a kid and I ran the streets and that is why it happened. This person took advantage. She said she was proud of me, that I did all right for a scared seven-year-old. I survived. I do feel really tired today. I took a short nap. I think it is the after-effects of theEMDR. I have to do more of them. This childhood stuff has to be dealt with on a new level. I have not run away. I believe this is going to help me. Today it is not important to dwell about the past pains in my life. It is important to finally let go of the abuse by healing the inner child with EMDR's I am growing; I am celebrating my 6th year, so how am I doing? I dealt with the breakup of my romantic relationship,with Nancy it ended in January. It has been 6 months, I have grown because of it, I was going out with Nancy for 17 months, I did pretty well. I realized I did nothing wrong she just ended it. I can live with it. I am going to therapy; I learned I am a co-dependent I am reading a book about that. I am a survivor of many kinds of abuse. As a child Iwas beaten, I was neglected I was given little emotional support. My parents never showed affection for each other I lived in a world of don't speak or show your emotions. It is a learning process to have a healthy relationship when you never had a role model I go to other meetings for all of these issues. I turned fifty this month, June 5. Rich Kane, the Bronx street kid, the juvenile delinquent, the dead-end kid, the motorcycle gang member. I did my time in county jails and prison. I saw the nuthouse and detox centers. I am doing all right. I work. I have my own place to live. I pay my bills on time. I have started to see this woman named Denise. She has depression. I am trying to learn about this illness. She is in the hospital right now. I went and saw her three times in the last week. I brought her flowers. Tuesday was my birthday. I was glad to see her. I have strong feelings for her. I have been seeing her for a month. We have only kissed a few times. I am going very slowly. I want to practice this intimacy on all levels. I really want to get to know her. I want her to get to know me. I am attracted to her. I do want to be with her in a more romantic way. I will wait. I have learned a lot about myself. I have grown. I have confidence in myself. I have self-worth; I have value. I am a decent and kind, loving human being. I do realize I want companionship. I am working on that. I have something to offer to someone. I am doing really well. My health is good. I am in remission over five years from the hepatitis C virus. I am really grateful for all of these miracles. I had a talk with Denise when she got out of the hospital. I told her I would just like to be her friend. I won't put any pressure on her. She needs a lot of extra help. . I am grateful to my higher power for all of my blessings and I hope Denise will find her way into recovery. Even though Nancy left me, I still look at it like a blessing. I will always love her because she was the first woman I ever fell in love with. She helped me get over the Hell's Angels. Now I am getting over her. I am doing really well. I am working. I have been in the union nineteen years. I am earning a decent living . I just turned fifty on June 5. I am in really good shape. I take pride in my daily exercise routine I am able to do thirteen hundred push-ups along with my weight lifting. I can still run up to two miles daily.. I have goals and dreams. Maybe someday I can go to Ireland for a visit. I have never been there. I dreamed of it when I was a kid. My family is from Limerick it would be nice to see where they came from. I am sober six years. What a miracle! I survived a murder attempt. I am a survivor. I keep trying to be a better person. I go to all kinds of meetings. I need the help. I am not ashamed to ask for it. I have a bunch of good friends in recovery. I have no romance in my life right now. That is all right; it will come again one day. I have learned to love and forgive others and myself. Anybody who reads my stuff has to understand that it helps me to stay sober. I tell my story as truthfully as I can recall. The truth sets me free. I am living a decent life now.

December 2007

To The High Bridge Horizon Newspaper.

To the people of The Bronx, NY. I grew up in High Bridge. We lived on Merriam Avenue. We had two apartments (1370 4th floor). We then moved to 1406 Merriam Ave on the 4th floor. We moved out in 1967, I was only 10 years old, I didn't like leaving. Anyway, I am now 50 years old. I am sober 6 and half years. I go to a lot of 12 steps meetings it is helping me get better. I just want to share some of my stories with you people although I don't blame my childhood, I do realize it did affect me, so here is what happened to me. My father was a violent drunk and hung out in all the bars on Ogden Ave. I used to go there looking for him. I got many beatings over the years, it would be impossible to count that high. I got used to the beatings. I use to like to run the streets and I had many accidents. I fell off the store roof on Ogden Avenue. Maybe I was 6 or 7. I hung out with the Moore twins, Kevin and Kenneth. They lived on Merriam Ave between 170 and 171 St. I also hung out with Ricky and Lonnie

Parker.. They lived on 170St. There father was a super in one the buildings.

We all ran the streets back then and we used to go down by the Harlem River under the High Bridge. We would swim and hang out. One day I was going down there, it was in the evening and I went looking for my friends. This man got a hold of me and took off my pants. He was behind me and it started to hurt. I didn't know what he was doing. The train came in, people got off. He held my mouth, he told me to shut up. No one had seen it, it was dark. He finished and then he let me go. I ran and I never said anything about this for over 40 years. A couple of years ago I wrote to a priest in Sacred Heart. He wrote back. He said the man stole my innocence, I never saw that person everagain. We moved out of the Bronx to Jersey. We ended up in Bergen Field and I started to drink when I was 11. I had a lot of problems with anger. I got into a lot of fights and I got into a lot of trouble.

I went away when I was 15 for burglary's and stolen cars. I did 18 months. I got into a lot of trouble over the years. I went away almost every year from the age of 15 to 28 years old, I did time in the County Jail in Bergen County. I also did time in Rikers.Island 10 months in 1980 or 81.

I also did state time in Jersey. I got two 5 year sentences for burglaries. I got one in 1975 and the other in 1980. I hit all the rehabs, detoxs and hospitals. Also the psyco wards. I drank a lot; I could drink over a half gallon of vodka a day. I lived in the streets for long periods of time in the 1970's and the 1980's. I remember going back to High Bridge when I was drunk in the 70's. The neighborhood was almost burned down. I remember being drunk and sleeping in one of the buildings. They were vacant, I didn't care. I hated myself for what I had become. I used to box when I was in jail and I lifted weights. I finally got off the streets. I stopped drinking for the first time in 1985. I stopped for over 12 years. I went back to the bottle in 1997.

When I wasn't drinking for the 12 years, I wasn't living the right kind of life. I rode with motorcycle gangs. I was still into violence. I rode with the Desperadoes M.C. we were out of the Bronx down by Arthur Ave near 188 St. I did leave them to prospect for the Hells Angels. I was voted in on July 31,1993. I wasn't drinking for 10 years in 1995. When a a rival gang in Jersey almost murdered me. Two people were in a car, they saw me on my bike and they followed me and pushed me into a parked car very hard and very fast. I was left for dead. I survived. I had to have leg surgery. The brothers in the Hells Angels were mad at me for this and later that year in October of 1995 I was kicked out. As I said I blame no one for any of this. I made the choices. They led me back to the bottle I am sober again. I am grateful to my higher power.for my second chance.

I have done all the things I didn't do the first time in my 12 step program. I got a sponsor. I read the big book. I have done the 12 steps to the best of my ability. I also attend therapy.along with my many meetings. . I pray daily for the strength to stay sober. I still go to the Bronx on my bike. There is a lot of new construction. High Bridge has turned around and it looks good. My life has turned around.

Thanks
Richard Kane

January 20th 2008

One year ago I was hurting, confused; my girfriend ended our relationship with no explanation. I did try to find out and I wanted another chance. It didn't happen I couldn't sleep I wasn't eating. I was working and going to meetings I talked about it I cried, I realized after several month there wasn't going to be another chance it took 5 or 6 months to get over this. Love can do that. I fell in love and I didn't realize it until it was over, love allows that I let the other person have her own life. I thought I did something wrong I know today that I didn't I was doing the best I could. She was only my 3rd girlfriend. I see the growth I am grateful for the time I spent with Nancy I was very new at romantic relationships, I didn't know what I was doing everything seemed alright Nancy always seemed happy. I learned I didn't know this person the way I thought I did. I got hurt, but I didn't get broken. I see now the wounded person that I am, I carried a lot of stuffed feelings from my childhood all of them came up and out because ofthe breakup. It was very painful for a while all of my childhood traumas were coming back. I was feeling the feelings. I was having flashbacks, I had some nightmares it seemed like my life was coming apart at the seams, I was very emotional I cried at some meetings this bothered me I felt weak almost cowardly. I started to relive the sex abuse. It seemed the more I worked on my recovery the harder it would get at times I started to get nightmares about it. Why now? Why after 40 years? I went and saw my mother and told her about the sex abuse, because she never knew. I was 7; I was amazed that she wanted to talk about her flowers or my younger brother Tom. She said "why didn't you tell your father? He would have killed the person". I told her I thought he would have killed me that's why I never said anything. She gave me some emotional support, I only stayed for an hour I went to a meeting in River Edge, and it was my friend Joe's anniversary. I asked to be the speaker for his anniversary and he let me.

I broke down and cried, I told the whole meeting about what happened with me and Nancy, and going to see my mother. I didn't tell my mother all the details. I told the meeting. I told them about the sexual abuse that happened as a child I went into more detail at the meeting than with my mother I only spoke about 10 or 15 minutes, I mostly talked about my childhood theses thoughts were coming back and they were very strong. I talked about some of the beatings I had gotten from my father, I remember telling them about getting a drawer smashed over my head, because the clothes weren't folded right. I recall speaking about the marching, the marine corp. hymn we had to sing . I remember when my father beat me with the hedge clippers; it was in Bergenfield, he beat me on the head with them. I had so many thoughts , all similar all violent. The violence that was done to me I spoke about them all, I finished my speaking commitment with all of the progress I have made in the last year. . I attend a weekly therapy meeting . I work with my therapist by doing EMDR's on my major traumas.. I continue attending many 12 step meetings These meetings are whats keeping me alive, today I have a future and it looks good. As for work

. I went back on January 2nd, I am in the laborers union 20 years, I got in 1988 I was sober 3 years I did something good for my self. I can see how much I have changed even though I didn't drink for over 12 years I can see I was only dry. I didn't have a sponsor back then but I do now. I wrote my fourth step and my life story. I pray everyday I believe in a higher power, I do the work. I leave the results in my higher powers hands the spirit guides the spirit provides God loves me and He will see me through, all things are possible with my higher Power. I am grateful to be alive and sober and healthy I love my higher power I love all the 12 step groups I go to and I love my self

January 2009

In August I was on my last week of unemployment I was #60 on the out of work list down at the union hall., Laborers local 592 Edgewater, NJ. I prayed to God to help me and he did. I got a call to go back to work at Giant stadium I got a job with Turn Key construction. It is a gift because the super and the 2 Foremen are in 12 step recovery. I am grateful for this, all the guys on the job made a donation for this Christmas party it is called Path of Hope, a non-profit organization I have been getting involved with. It is run by a bunch of people helping underprivileged children with holiday parties and summer camps . I helped out this year. It was on Saturday December 13th it was the 1st time I ever did something like this. We gave toys and bicycles to 50 families that don't have anything. It opened my eyes, I was able to see how big of a difference stuff like this could make. I plan on doing it again this year, I am still working for Turn Key I am a good laborer I am proud to be a member of local 592 in NJ. I am sober and I am grateful. Everyone is waiting for my book, people on the job, people in all of the 12 step recovery meetings, it is a miracle the Bronx street kid is now an author I hope my book helps others I am doing alright I am single I am not seeing anyone today I am hopeful to have companionship when the time is right . I am still in group therapy I attend recovery meetings almost every night,I sing in a choir today and I found I am not bad at drawing. Not bad for someone who use to sleep in the gutter. I practice affirmations, such as every day in every way I am getting better,better and better, I surrender to the spirit and let the spirit guide me. I believe in my self when I let go of the old life, I make room for the new life. I pray for health and harmony for everybody. I have been blessed with recovery; I have learned to forgive others I have prayed for all the people who caused me harm. I am grateful to God for seeing something worthwhile in me. I still go to a group called hopes I go there for the sex abuse I am no longer ashamed or guilty about this I have been set free I am grateful to my higher power who loves and accepts me as I am. I am learning to do the same.

Sincerely yours, Rich Kane

Affirmation

January 12, 2008

I accept myself hear and now. I am now willing to experience all my feelings. I enjoy being sober. I love my freedom. God is the unlimited source of my supply. Grace is acceptance of the love of God. Love will enter immediately into any mind that wants it. See the love of God in me and I will see it everywhere. Love can live only in peace. Learn how to look on all things with love appreciation and open mind ness. Light and joy and peace abide in me. I am one with God. Peace to my brothers and sisters who are one with me. Do you want peace? Forgiveness offers it. Forgiveness is the key to happiness. Forgive the past and let it go for it is gone Peace can be found only through complete forgiveness. I am free today. I am no longer held captive by the pain of my past. Restoration means I bring them to the one that is able to heal them. I was wounded I needed to be restored, I asked for enlightenment. It is only through exposure that I can begin to face what happened in my past and move on with the healing. Will I allow the Spirit to begin to expose these troubled areas? Will I allow his light to heal those hurts? Will I let him set me free? I allow the Spirit to work through me and guide me I am blessed with abundance. The 12 steps have set me free. They are a group of principles, which if practiced as a

way of life can expel the obsession to drink. I thank God for these miracles.

Affirmations

Febuary 24th 2008

Knowing how another human being lives and functions on the inside .How he or she handles the vicissitudes of life copes with it joys and frustrations, faces critical choices meets failure and defeat as well as challenge and success – is what enables us to feel prepared for life, the availability of appropriate people with whom we can identify. A man walking through the forest saw a fox that had lost its legs and wondered how it lived. Then he saw a tiger come up with game in its mouth, the tiger ate his fill and left the rest of the meat for the fox, the next day God fed the fox by means of the same tiger The man began to wonder at

God's greatness and said to himself I too shall rest in the corner with full trust in the Lord and He will provide. He did this for many days but nothing happened He was close to death when he heard a voice say "O You who are on the path of error open your eyes to the truth ,stop imitating the disabled fox and follow the example of the tiger.

March 5th 2008

What could you want forgiveness cannot give.Do you want peace forgiveness offers it.

Do you want happiness , a quit mind, a certainty of purpose and a sense of worth and beauty

That transcends the world? Do you want care and safety, and the warmth of sure protection always? Do you want a quietness that cannot be disturbed, a gentleness that never can be hurt,

A deep abiding comfort and a rest so perfect it can never be upset? All this forgiveness offers you. forgiveness is the key to happiness Here is the answer to your search for peace, here is the key to meaning in a world that seems to make no sense, here is the way to safety in apparent dangers that appear to threaten you at every turn and bring uncertainty to all your hope's of ever finding quietness and peace. Here all questions are answered,here the end of all uncertainty ensured at last.Forgive the past and let it go,for it is gone.You who want peace can find it only by complete forgiveness.

March 7ᵗʰ 2008

Hope is born while facing the unknown and discovering that one is not alone .I thank God and recovery for my sobriety. There is a God and I am not it .I must learn to listen and listen to learn. I have to remain teachable .Spirituality is one of those realities that we have only so long as we seek it, as soon as we stop seeking we stop finding As soon as we think we got it we most certainly lost it .The twelve steps are a group of principles, spiritual in there nature , which, if practiced as a way of life, can expel the obsession to drink and enable the suffer to become happily and usefully whole. Keep it simple utilize don't analyze Know God ,know peace I trust my higher power with everything.

May 27, 2008

Everyone wants the kind of love I have to offer. I am wonderfully loving I heal the world with my love.God is the strength in which I trust. There is nothing to fear. I commit to honor, obey and love and cherish my own being My commitment is to truth and honesty If you love yourself others will love you if you respect yourself others will respect you. If you trust yourself others will trust you. If you are gentle and compassionate with yourself others will treat you with compassion. If you appreciate yourself others will appreciate you I live sober I live one day at a time I do one thing at a time and I take one step at a time.

June 20 2008

If God is for me who could be against me Replace the negative with the positive. To the taker an empty life,to the giver a full life Big ego big problems no ego no problems When I let go of the old life I make room for the new life, spirit guides ,spirit provides. I allow peace, love and harmony into my life,I also want all of these blessings for everybody .Love covers a multitude of sins.

All of these affirmations help me to stay sober and become a better person one day at a time

MAR 1 0

LaVergne, TN USA
17 February 2010
173319LV00001B/99/P